Section One: Chemotherapy Calendar.

A place to plan out your treatments.

Chemotherapy Plan

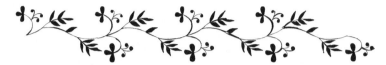

Month: _____

Monday	Tuesday	Wednesday	Thursday	Friday	Saturday	Sunday

_____

_____

Chemotherapy Plan

Month: _____

Monday	Tuesday	Wednesday	Thursday	Friday	Saturday	Sunday

_____

_____

Chemotherapy Plan

Month: _____

Monday	Tuesday	Wednesday	Thursday	Friday	Saturday	Sunday

_____

_____

Chemotherapy Plan

Month: _____

Monday	Tuesday	Wednesday	Thursday	Friday	Saturday	Sunday

_____

_____

Chemotherapy Plan

Month: _____

Monday	Tuesday	Wednesday	Thursday	Friday	Saturday	Sunday

_____

_____

Chemotherapy Plan

Month: _____

Monday	Tuesday	Wednesday	Thursday	Friday	Saturday	Sunday

_____

_____

Chemotherapy Plan

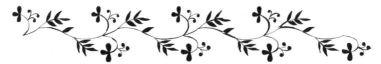

Month: _____

Monday	Tuesday	Wednesday	Thursday	Friday	Saturday	Sunday

_____

_____

Chemotherapy Plan

Month: _____

Monday	Tuesday	Wednesday	Thursday	Friday	Saturday	Sunday

_____

_____

Chemotherapy Plan

Month: _____

Monday	Tuesday	Wednesday	Thursday	Friday	Saturday	Sunday

_____

_____

Chemotherapy Plan

Month: _____

Monday	Tuesday	Wednesday	Thursday	Friday	Saturday	Sunday

_____

_____

Chemotherapy Plan

Month: _____

Monday	Tuesday	Wednesday	Thursday	Friday	Saturday	Sunday

_____

_____

Medication List

Medication List

Medication List

Notes about my Scans

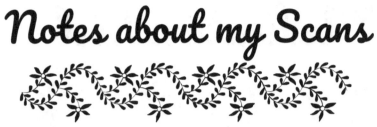

Scan Date: _____

Scan Type: _____

Scan Results Expected When?:

_____

My Next Appointment:

_____

Scan Results:

_____

_____

_____

_____

Notes about my Scans

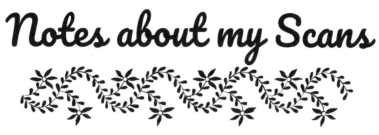

Scan Date: _____

Scan Type: _____

Scan Results Expected When?:

_____

My Next Appointment:

_____

Scan Results:

_____

_____

_____

_____

Notes about my Scans

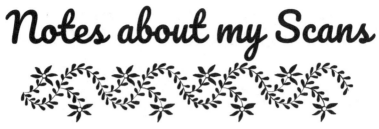

Scan Date: ———————————————

Scan Type: ———————————————

Scan Results Expected When?:

———————————————

My Next Appointment:

———————————————

Scan Results:

———————————————

———————————————

———————————————

———————————————

Notes about my Scans

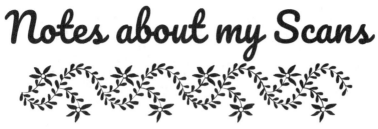

Scan Date: _____

Scan Type: _____

Scan Results Expected When?:

_____

My Next Appointment:

_____

Scan Results:

_____

_____

_____

_____

Notes about my Scans

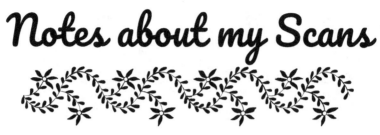

Scan Date: _____

Scan Type: _____

Scan Results Expected When?:

_____

My Next Appointment:

_____

Scan Results:

_____

_____

_____

_____

Notes about my Scans

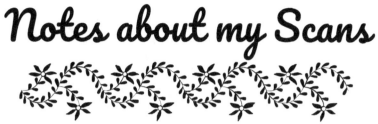

Scan Date: _____

Scan Type: _____

Scan Results Expected When?:

_____

My Next Appointment:

_____

Scan Results:

_____

_____

_____

_____

Notes about my Scans

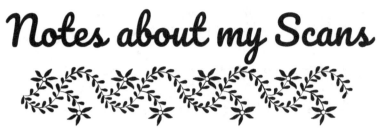

Scan Date: _____

Scan Type: _____

Scan Results Expected When?:

_____

My Next Appointment:

_____

Scan Results:

_____

_____

_____

_____

Notes about my Scans

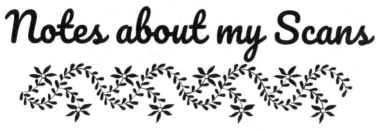

Scan Date: _____

Scan Type: _____

Scan Results Expected When?:

_____

My Next Appointment:

_____

Scan Results:

_____

_____

_____

_____

Chemo Number One

Did you meet with the oncologist today?

Yes ☐ No ☐

Date: _____

Notes from your appointment:

My Blood Counts:

_____

_____

_____

_____

_____

Pre-Meds Given Today:

_____

_____

_____

_____

_____

Chemo Drugs Given Today:

_____

_____

_____

_____

_____

Any side effects during the infusion?

_____

_____

_____

_____

_____

Water Tracker:

How is my mood?

_____

_____

_____

_____

_____

Side Effects Experienced Post Chemo:

○ _____

○ _____

○ _____

○ _____

○ _____

Meds Taken to Manage:

○ _____

○ _____

○ _____

○ _____

○ _____

○ _____

Side Effects Experienced Post Chemo:

○ _____
○ _____
○ _____
○ _____
○ _____

Meds Taken to Manage:

○ _____
○ _____
○ _____
○ _____
○ _____
○ _____

Notes to go over with my oncologist:

○ _____

○ _____

○ _____

○ _____

○ _____

○ _____

○ _____

○ _____

○ _____

○ _____

○ _____

Chemo Number Two

Did you meet with the oncologist today?

Yes ☐   No ☐

Date: _____

Notes from your appointment:

My Blood Counts:

_____

_____

_____

_____

_____

Pre-Meds Given Today:

_____

_____

_____

_____

_____

Chemo Drugs Given Today:

_____

_____

_____

_____

_____

Any side effects during the infusion?

_____

_____

_____

_____

_____

Water Tracker:

How is my mood?

_____

_____

_____

_____

_____

Side Effects Experienced
Post Chemo:

O _____

O _____

O _____

O _____

O _____

Meds Taken to Manage:

O _____

O _____

O _____

O _____

O _____

O _____

Side Effects Experienced Post Chemo:

- ○ _____
- ○ _____
- ○ _____
- ○ _____
- ○ _____

Meds Taken to Manage:

- ○ _____
- ○ _____
- ○ _____
- ○ _____
- ○ _____
- ○ _____

Notes to go over with my oncologist:

- ○ _____
- ○ _____
- ○ _____
- ○ _____
- ○ _____
- ○ _____
- ○ _____
- ○ _____
- ○ _____
- ○ _____

Chemo Number Three

Did you meet with the oncologist today?

Yes ☐ No ☐

Date: _____

Notes from your appointment:

My Blood Counts:

_____

_____

_____

_____

_____

Pre-Meds Given Today:

_____

_____

_____

_____

_____

Chemo Drugs Given Today:

_____

_____

_____

_____

_____

Any side effects during the infusion?

_____

_____

_____

_____

_____

Water Tracker:

How is my mood?

_____

_____

_____

_____

_____

Side Effects Experienced Post Chemo:

○ _____
○ _____
○ _____
○ _____
○ _____

Meds Taken to Manage:

○ _____
○ _____
○ _____
○ _____
○ _____
○ _____

Side Effects Experienced Post Chemo:

- ○ _____
- ○ _____
- ○ _____
- ○ _____
- ○ _____

Meds Taken to Manage:

- ○ _____
- ○ _____
- ○ _____
- ○ _____
- ○ _____
- ○ _____

Notes to go over with my oncologist:

- ○ _____
- ○ _____
- ○ _____
- ○ _____
- ○ _____
- ○ _____
- ○ _____
- ○ _____
- ○ _____
- ○ _____
- ○ _____

Chemo Number Four

Did you meet with the oncologist today?

Yes ☐ No ☐

Date: _____

Notes from your appointment:

My Blood Counts:

_____

_____

_____

_____

_____

Pre-Meds Given Today:

_____

_____

_____

_____

_____

Chemo Drugs Given Today:

_____

_____

_____

_____

_____

Any side effects during the infusion?

_____

_____

_____

_____

_____

Water Tracker:

How is my mood?

_____

_____

_____

_____

_____

Side Effects Experienced Post Chemo:

○ _____

○ _____

○ _____

○ _____

○ _____

Meds Taken to Manage:

○ _____

○ _____

○ _____

○ _____

○ _____

○ _____

Side Effects Experienced Post Chemo:

○ _____

○ _____

○ _____

○ _____

○ _____

Meds Taken to Manage:

○ _____

○ _____

○ _____

○ _____

○ _____

○ _____

Notes to go over with my oncologist:

- _____
- _____
- _____
- _____
- _____
- _____
- _____
- _____
- _____
- _____
- _____

Chemo Number Five

Did you meet with the oncologist today?

Yes ☐ No ☐

Date: _____

Notes from your appointment:

My Blood Counts:

_____

_____

_____

_____

Pre-Meds Given Today:

_____

_____

_____

_____

Chemo Drugs Given Today:

_____

_____

_____

_____

Any side effects during the infusion?

_____

_____

_____

_____

_____

Water Tracker:

How is my mood?

_____

_____

_____

_____

_____

Side Effects Experienced
Post Chemo:

○ _____

○ _____

○ _____

○ _____

○ _____

Meds Taken to Manage:

○ _____

○ _____

○ _____

○ _____

○ _____

○ _____

Side Effects Experienced Post Chemo:

- ○ _____
- ○ _____
- ○ _____
- ○ _____
- ○ _____

Meds Taken to Manage:

- ○ _____
- ○ _____
- ○ _____
- ○ _____
- ○ _____
- ○ _____

Notes to go over with my oncologist:

○ _____

○ _____

○ _____

○ _____

○ _____

○ _____

○ _____

○ _____

○ _____

○ _____

○ _____

Chemo Number Six

Did you meet with the oncologist today?

Yes ☐ No ☐

Date: _____

Notes from your appointment:

My Blood Counts:

_____

_____

_____

_____

_____

Pre-Meds Given Today:

_____

_____

_____

_____

_____

Chemo Drugs Given Today:

_____

_____

_____

_____

_____

Any side effects during the infusion?

_____

_____

_____

_____

_____

Water Tracker:

How is my mood?

_____

_____

_____

_____

_____

Side Effects Experienced Post Chemo:

○ _____

○ _____

○ _____

○ _____

○ _____

Meds Taken to Manage:

○ _____

○ _____

○ _____

○ _____

○ _____

○ _____

Side Effects Experienced Post Chemo:

○ _____

○ _____

○ _____

○ _____

○ _____

Meds Taken to Manage:

○ _____

○ _____

○ _____

○ _____

○ _____

○ _____

Notes to go over with my oncologist:

- ○ _____
- ○ _____
- ○ _____
- ○ _____
- ○ _____
- ○ _____
- ○ _____
- ○ _____
- ○ _____
- ○ _____
- ○ _____

Chemo Number Seven

Did you meet with the oncologist today?

Yes ☐ No ☐

Date: _____

Notes from your appointment:

My Blood Counts:

_____

_____

_____

_____

_____

Pre-Meds Given Today:

_____

_____

_____

_____

_____

Chemo Drugs Given Today:

_____

_____

_____

_____

_____

Any side effects during the infusion?

_____

_____

_____

_____

_____

Water Tracker:

How is my mood?

_____

_____

_____

_____

_____

Side Effects Experienced Post Chemo:

- _____
- _____
- _____
- _____
- _____

Meds Taken to Manage:

- _____
- _____
- _____
- _____
- _____
- _____

Side Effects Experienced Post Chemo:

○ _____

○ _____

○ _____

○ _____

○ _____

Meds Taken to Manage:

○ _____

○ _____

○ _____

○ _____

○ _____

○ _____

Notes to go over with my oncologist:

- _____
- _____
- _____
- _____
- _____
- _____
- _____
- _____
- _____
- _____
- _____

Chemo Number Eight

Did you meet with the oncologist today?

Yes ☐ No ☐

Date: _____

Notes from your appointment:

My Blood Counts:

_____

_____

_____

_____

Pre-Meds Given Today:

_____

_____

_____

_____

Chemo Drugs Given Today:

_____

_____

_____

_____

Any side effects during the infusion?

_____

_____

_____

_____

_____

Water Tracker:

How is my mood?

_____

_____

_____

_____

_____

Side Effects Experienced
Post Chemo:

○ _____

○ _____

○ _____

○ _____

○ _____

Meds Taken to Manage:

○ _____

○ _____

○ _____

○ _____

○ _____

○ _____

Side Effects Experienced Post Chemo:

- ○ _____
- ○ _____
- ○ _____
- ○ _____
- ○ _____

Meds Taken to Manage:

- ○ _____
- ○ _____
- ○ _____
- ○ _____
- ○ _____
- ○ _____

Notes to go over with my oncologist:

○ _____
○ _____
○ _____
○ _____
○ _____
○ _____
○ _____
○ _____
○ _____
○ _____
○ _____

Chemo Number Nine

Did you meet with the oncologist today?

Yes ☐ No ☐

Date: _____

Notes from your appointment:

My Blood Counts:

_____

_____

_____

_____

_____

Pre-Meds Given Today:

_____

_____

_____

_____

_____

Chemo Drugs Given Today:

_____

_____

_____

_____

_____

Any side effects during the infusion?

_____

_____

_____

_____

_____

Water Tracker:

How is my mood?

_____

_____

_____

_____

_____

Side Effects Experienced
Post Chemo:

○ _____

○ _____

○ _____

○ _____

○ _____

Meds Taken to Manage:

○ _____

○ _____

○ _____

○ _____

○ _____

○ _____

Side Effects Experienced Post Chemo:

○ _____

○ _____

○ _____

○ _____

○ _____

Meds Taken to Manage:

○ _____

○ _____

○ _____

○ _____

○ _____

○ _____

Notes to go over with my oncologist:

- ○ _____
- ○ _____
- ○ _____
- ○ _____
- ○ _____
- ○ _____
- ○ _____
- ○ _____
- ○ _____
- ○ _____
- ○ _____

Chemo Number Ten

Did you meet with the oncologist today?

Yes ☐ No ☐

Date: _____

Notes from your appointment:

My Blood Counts:

Pre-Meds Given Today:

Chemo Drugs Given Today:

Any side effects during the infusion?

_____

_____

_____

_____

_____

Water Tracker:

How is my mood?

_____

_____

_____

_____

_____

Side Effects Experienced Post Chemo:

- ○ _____
- ○ _____
- ○ _____
- ○ _____
- ○ _____

Meds Taken to Manage:

- ○ _____
- ○ _____
- ○ _____
- ○ _____
- ○ _____
- ○ _____

Side Effects Experienced Post Chemo:

○ _____

○ _____

○ _____

○ _____

○ _____

Meds Taken to Manage:

○ _____

○ _____

○ _____

○ _____

○ _____

○ _____

Notes to go over with my oncologist:

○ _____

○ _____

○ _____

○ _____

○ _____

○ _____

○ _____

○ _____

○ _____

○ _____

○ _____

Chemo Number Eleven

Did you meet with the oncologist today?

Yes ☐   No ☐

Date: _____

Notes from your appointment:

My Blood Counts:

_____

_____

_____

_____

Pre-Meds Given Today:

_____

_____

_____

_____

Chemo Drugs Given Today:

_____

_____

_____

_____

Any side effects during the infusion?

_____

_____

_____

_____

_____

Water Tracker:

How is my mood?

_____

_____

_____

_____

_____

Side Effects Experienced
Post Chemo:

○ _____

○ _____

○ _____

○ _____

○ _____

Meds Taken to Manage:

○ _____

○ _____

○ _____

○ _____

○ _____

○ _____

Side Effects Experienced Post Chemo:

- ○ _____
- ○ _____
- ○ _____
- ○ _____
- ○ _____

Meds Taken to Manage:

- ○ _____
- ○ _____
- ○ _____
- ○ _____
- ○ _____
- ○ _____

Notes to go over with my oncologist:

- _____
- _____
- _____
- _____
- _____
- _____
- _____
- _____
- _____
- _____
- _____

Chemo Number Twelve

Did you meet with the oncologist today?

Yes ☐ No ☐

Date: _____

Notes from your appointment:

My Blood Counts:

_____

_____

_____

_____

_____

Pre-Meds Given Today:

_____

_____

_____

_____

_____

Chemo Drugs Given Today:

_____

_____

_____

_____

_____

Any side effects during the infusion?

_____

_____

_____

_____

_____

Water Tracker:

How is my mood?

_____

_____

_____

_____

_____

Side Effects Experienced Post Chemo:

○ _____
○ _____
○ _____
○ _____
○ _____

Meds Taken to Manage:

○ _____
○ _____
○ _____
○ _____
○ _____
○ _____

Side Effects Experienced Post Chemo:

- ○ _____
- ○ _____
- ○ _____
- ○ _____
- ○ _____

Meds Taken to Manage:

- ○ _____
- ○ _____
- ○ _____
- ○ _____
- ○ _____
- ○ _____

Notes to go over with my oncologist:

- _____
- _____
- _____
- _____
- _____
- _____
- _____
- _____
- _____
- _____
- _____

Chemo Number Thirteen

Did you meet with the oncologist today?

Yes ☐ No ☐

Date: —————————————————

Notes from your appointment:

My Blood Counts:

_____

_____

_____

_____

Pre-Meds Given Today:

_____

_____

_____

_____

Chemo Drugs Given Today:

_____

_____

_____

_____

Any side effects during the infusion?

_____

_____

_____

_____

_____

Water Tracker:

How is my mood?

_____

_____

_____

_____

_____

Side Effects Experienced Post Chemo:

○ _____

○ _____

○ _____

○ _____

○ _____

Meds Taken to Manage:

○ _____

○ _____

○ _____

○ _____

○ _____

○ _____

Side Effects Experienced Post Chemo:

- ○ _____
- ○ _____
- ○ _____
- ○ _____
- ○ _____

Meds Taken to Manage:

- ○ _____
- ○ _____
- ○ _____
- ○ _____
- ○ _____
- ○ _____

Notes to go over with my oncologist:

- ○ _____
- ○ _____
- ○ _____
- ○ _____
- ○ _____
- ○ _____
- ○ _____
- ○ _____
- ○ _____
- ○ _____
- ○ _____

Chemo Number Fourteen

※※ ※※ ※※ ※※ ※※

Did you meet with the oncologist today?

Yes ☐ No ☐

Date: _____

Notes from your appointment:

My Blood Counts:

_____

_____

_____

_____

_____

Pre-Meds Given Today:

_____

_____

_____

_____

_____

Chemo Drugs Given Today:

_____

_____

_____

_____

_____

Any side effects during the infusion?

_____

_____

_____

_____

_____

Water Tracker:

How is my mood?

_____

_____

_____

_____

_____

Side Effects Experienced Post Chemo:

- ○ _____
- ○ _____
- ○ _____
- ○ _____
- ○ _____

Meds Taken to Manage:

- ○ _____
- ○ _____
- ○ _____
- ○ _____
- ○ _____
- ○ _____

Side Effects Experienced Post Chemo:

- ○ _____
- ○ _____
- ○ _____
- ○ _____
- ○ _____

Meds Taken to Manage:

- ○ _____
- ○ _____
- ○ _____
- ○ _____
- ○ _____
- ○ _____

Notes to go over with my oncologist:

○ _____

○ _____

○ _____

○ _____

○ _____

○ _____

○ _____

○ _____

○ _____

○ _____

○ _____

Chemo Number Fifteen

Did you meet with the oncologist today?

Yes ☐ No ☐

Date: _____

Notes from your appointment:

My Blood Counts:

_____

_____

_____

_____

Pre-Meds Given Today:

_____

_____

_____

_____

Chemo Drugs Given Today:

_____

_____

_____

_____

Any side effects during the infusion?

_____

_____

_____

_____

Water Tracker:

How is my mood?

_____

_____

_____

_____

_____

Side Effects Experienced Post Chemo:

○ _____

○ _____

○ _____

○ _____

○ _____

Meds Taken to Manage:

○ _____

○ _____

○ _____

○ _____

○ _____

○ _____

Side Effects Experienced Post Chemo:

○ _____

○ _____

○ _____

○ _____

○ _____

Meds Taken to Manage:

○ _____

○ _____

○ _____

○ _____

○ _____

○ _____

Notes to go over with my oncologist:

- ○ _____
- ○ _____
- ○ _____
- ○ _____
- ○ _____
- ○ _____
- ○ _____
- ○ _____
- ○ _____
- ○ _____
- ○ _____

Notes

Notes

Notes

Notes

Notes

Notes

Made in the USA
Middletown, DE
25 May 2022